100 Questions Psychiatry Should Face

100 Questions Psychiatry Should Face

Avery Z. Conner

Writers Club Press
New York Lincoln Shanghai

100 Questions Psychiatry Should Face

Writers Club Press
an imprint of iUniverse, Inc.

For information address:
iUniverse, Inc.
2021 Pine Lake Road, Suite 100
Lincoln, NE 68512
www.iuniverse.com

ISBN: 0-595-26294-5

Printed in the United States of America

Contents

Introduction

In the last fifty years, psychiatry has been transformed largely by the advent and increasing availability of mood altering medications. These medications have focused attention on the biochemical aspects of psychiatric disorders, and perhaps less emphasis has been placed on talk therapy. Medicinal treatment of psychiatric disorders remains largely subjective—based both on the impressions of the physician and the self-reported symptoms of the patient. So the physician makes an educated guess about which medication to try and how large the dose should be, and then waits, often for more than two weeks, for the subjective outcome. Unfortunately, subjective, trial and error treatment methods often lead to inadequate treatment. Therefore, a new psychiatry is needed that rigorously applies the scientific method to improve treatment by generating testable theories and rigorously gathering both objective data, and when necessary subjective data, to test those theories. A reasonable theory is better than no theory at all for at least two reasons: 1) it affirms or eliminates one of the possibilities, and 2) it stimulates discussion. Also, a proactive approach is needed to determine which new drugs, with which new mechanisms of action, are needed to more effectively treat mental illness, rather than just "listening" to the effects of drugs after they're available. The question is not can psychiatry be changed, because it can, but in what ways, if any, should it be. For example, should we be dissecting personality and mental illness to the nth degree? Maybe all that knowledge is going to screw up the experience of being human. And one can make the argument that we shouldn't interfere with nature, and that can be said about all of healthcare, but on the other hand maybe it is a basic part of human nature to figure out ways to heal the body. The argument can also be made that society is becoming increasingly unnatural, which causes more mental illness, and therefore we must create something unnatural (namely medications) to combat this. So some of the challenges we face to improve psychiatry are: to make better use of the existing medications, to create better medications with more specific actions and fewer side effects, to use talk therapy more effectively, and to change our lifestyles.

1

The Big Three Neurotransmitters

o o o o o o o o o o o o o o o o o o o o o o o o o o o o o o o o

I refer to the neurotransmitters serotonin, norepinephrine, and dopamine as the "Big Three" because all existing antidepressants and mood stabilizers with known mechanisms of action are thought to achieve their effects on mood by affecting one or more of them.

Question 1

Can abnormalities of one or more of the Big Three neurotransmitter systems explain every type of mental illness?

Theory: No.

Question 2

When one of the Big Three neurotransmitter levels is altered by an antidepressant or mood stabilizer, is personality altered?

Note: Psychiatrist Peter Kramer discusses this subject in his landmark book, *Listening to Prozac*.

Question 3

Which aspects of mood does each of the Big Three neurotransmitter systems affect? Which aspects of emotion? Which aspects of thought? Which aspects of sensation? And are mood, emotion, thought, and sensation neurochemically independent of each other?

Question 4

In what ways, if any, do the Big Three neurotransmitter systems interact with each other? For example, if a medication alters the level of one of the Big Three, do the levels of the other two change? If so, is the recruitment continuous or is there a threshold?

Theory: When either serotonin or norepinephrine increases, dopamine also increases. This theory is derived from the observation that different antidepressants that boost either serotonin or norepinephrine can each induce mania, which probably results from the recruitment of dopamine.

Question 5

By what means does the brain regulate the level of each of the Big Three neurotransmitters? For example, when one of the Big Three gets to a threshold level, does the brain have a feedback mechanism that brings the neurotransmitter back to its normal level? Moreover, is the feedback mechanism continuous or thresholded?

Question 6

In an unmedicated individual, are the levels of each of the Big Three neurotransmitters independent of each other?

Theory: No, people high in either serotonin or norepinephrine or both are also high in dopamine.

Question 7

Does serotonin form a sensory-cognitive-emotional filter? If so, does serotonin convey pure attenuation of the senses, thoughts, and emotions or also alteration of them?

Note: Many researchers believe serotonin serves as a barrier against stress, so perhaps it does so by affecting the senses, thoughts, and emotions. And serotonin is distributed within the sensory, cognitive, and emotional regions of the brain.

Question 8

Does serotonin affect the traits listed in Peter Kramer's *Listening to Prozac*: compulsion, sensitivity, risk, self-esteem, ability to experience pleasure, (and stress tolerance)?

Theory: It affects each of these traits.

Question 9

Does norepinephrine also affect sensory-cognitive-emotional sensitivity?

Note: Norepinephrine is distributed within the sensory, cognitive, and emotional regions of the brain.

Question 10

Does dopamine affect the speed of thought and the ability to experience pleasure?

Note: Dopamine is distributed densely in the prefrontal region of the brain (thought to be involved in thinking) as well as in the emotional regions of the brain.

Question 11

What engineering principles can be applied to understanding how the Big Three neurotransmitter systems operate in the brain?

Note: Whether one believes the brain was engineered by evolution or some other creative force, engineering principles probably apply to its operations, such as positive/negative feedback regulation.

Question 12

Should much of the fundamental treatment of mental illness focus on adjusting the balance of serotonin and norepinephrine in the brain?

Theory: Depression, bipolar disorder, and schizophrenia each involve disturbances of one or both of these two neurotransmitter systems.

Question 13

Do the Big Three neurotransmitters have a steady baseline output in the synapse or can they be briefly pulsed out as well in response to environmental stimuli?

Theory: Dopamine can be pulsed out in the pleasure region of the brain, but it only seeps out at a baseline rate in the thinking region of the brain. Serotonin and norepinephrine only seep out at a baseline rate.

Question 14

Can the Big Three neurotransmitter systems change in a sustained manner based on external circumstances, to better adapt the individual for new circumstances, such as dominance?

Theory: In humans, only dopamine adapts to external circumstances in a novelty dependent manner, with greater novelty releasing greater dopamine.

Question 15

To what extent do the Big Three neurotransmitter systems affect athletic performance?

Theory: Serotonin enhances explosive movements, whereas norepinephrine enhances sustained movements.

Note: In animals that live in social groups that have dominance hierarchies, the "alpha" animal, who usually has the highest serotonin level, tends to win aggressive conflicts.

Question 16

If the Big Three neurotransmitter systems affect athletic performance, then do they also affect taste preference, and therefore preference for intake of certain types of foods?

Theory: People with high serotonin tend to prefer foods that enhance explosive movements, whereas people with high norepinephrine tend to prefer foods that enhance sustained movements.

Question 17

What is the relationship between sexual orientation and the Big Three neurotransmitter systems?

Theory: Heterosexual men tend to be high in serotonin, low in norepinephrine, whereas homosexual men tend to be high in norepinephrine, low in serotonin. Heterosexual women tend to be high in norepinephrine, low in serotonin, whereas homosexual women tend to be high in serotonin, low in norepinephrine.

Note: A lower serotonin level may explain why more women than men are diagnosed with depression.

Question 18

What is the relationship between the Big Three neurotransmitter systems and intelligence?

Theory: People high in serotonin tend to have instinctive intelligence, whereas people low in serotonin tend to have technical intelligence.

Question 19

Are mood, emotion, thought, and sensation affected by any neurotransmitter system other than the Big Three?

Note: GABA, glutamate, acetylcholine and other neurotransmitters may also affect these entities.

Theory: Acetylcholine is most similar in its brain distribution to the Big Three, so it may also affect these entities.

Question 20

To what extent do we need to understand the details of the Big Three neurotransmitter systems in order to understand mental illness?

Note: The Big Three are distributed in different areas of the brain, in circuits within areas (cortical layers), have subtypes of receptors that may include different circuits, and there may be long-term molecular changes as a result of the Big Three binding to their receptors (such as growth of dendritic spines, cell death/birth, changes in receptor densities, and other synaptic plasticities).

Question 21

Is the part of the serotonin and norepinephrine systems that is relevant to mood their diffuse connections with the sensory regions of the brain or their localized connections with the emotional regions of the brain? Or both?

Theory: Only the connections with the emotional regions of the brain affect mood.

Question 22

Will the distribution of receptor subtypes in the brain, in the foreseeable future when medications are the principal treatment available, set the limits on the specificity of psychopharmacology? And how many receptor subtypes remain to be discovered?

Question 23

Is there an optimal operating level range for each of the Big Three neurotransmitters, such that there is mental disturbance both when one is too low and when one is too high?

Theory: Yes.

Question 24

Do many people have a serotonin deficiency? Is it healthy to have as much serotonin as possible, or is too much of it unhealthy?

Note: A prevailing view is that many people are deficient in serotonin, but perhaps this is not the case. Moreover, a common view is that the more serotonin one has, the happier one is, and perhaps this is not the case.

Question 25

What is the relationship, if any, between sickness/fever and the Big Three neurotransmitter systems?

Note: Some people describe depression as a feverlike state, so perhaps the feeling of being sick is mediated by one or more of the Big Three.

Question 26

What is the relationship between the Big Three neurotransmitter systems and body temperature?

Note: The street drug ecstasy, which is thought to act on the Big Three, affects body temperature.

Question 27

In what manner are the genetics of the Big Three neurotransmitter systems transmitted from parents to their children?

Theory: Genetic transmission of serotonin and norepinephrine genes is "sign-preserving" between a parent and child of the same sex, whereas transmission is "sign-reversing" between a parent and child of the opposite sex. In other words, if a mother is high in norepinephrine and low in serotonin, and her children inherit the mother's serotonin and norepinephrine level determining genes, her female children will tend to be high norepinephrine and low in serotonin, whereas her male children will tend to be low in norepinephrine and high in serotonin.

2

Depression and Mania

Question 28

In a given depressed individual, is the level of one or more of the Big Three neurotransmitters lower than the normal level in that individual?

Theory: Yes.

Question 29

In a given manic individual, is the level of one or more of the Big Three neurotransmitters higher than the normal level in that individual?

Theory: Dopamine is always abnormally high during mania, as a result of feedforward input from an abnormally high level of serotonin or norepinephrine or both.

Question 30

Do bipolar individuals have the set point of one or more of the Big Three neurotransmitter systems beyond the threshold for mania during the normal (default) state? Or instead are the regulatory systems messed up such that oscillation of mood occurs?

Note: Maybe once oscillations occur, set point is disturbed or nonexistent.

Question 31

Why is bipolar disorder a predictor of wealth?

Note: For a discussion of this subject, see Goodwin and Jamison's *Manic-Depressive Illness.*

Question 32

Is there a neurochemical threshold for depression or mania or is it continuous?

Theory: It is continuous, with some thresholds, such as a neurochemical disturbance causing premature awakening.

Question 33

To what extent can so-called situational depression manifest itself neurochemically? Is one form of depression the result of severe dopaminergic adaptation to the environment?

Theory: Yes.

Question 34

Are there different types of depressions (perhaps beyond the atypical/typical dichotomy) and manias with different underlying Big Three neurotransmitter system abnormalities, that should be treated with different medicinal regimens? Is the atypical depression (oversleeping and overeating) and typical depression (undersleeping and undereating) dichotomy real or an oversimplification?

Theory: There are different types of depressions, with different underlying Big Three abnormalities, and two examples are atypical and typical depressions. Perhaps atypical depression involves low serotonin, whereas typical depression involves low norepinephrine.

Question 35

To what extent can the individual affect the cycling of his mood? In particular, can the individual push himself for a number of days and then cause a subsequent depression?

Note: Sleep deprivation can induce mania.

Question 36

What is the relationship between the Big Three neurotransmitter systems and sleep disturbance?

Note: Mania and depression are almost always accompanied by sleep disturbance.

Question 37

Under what circumstances does healing of the brain from a manic or depressive episode occur? When, if ever, is irreversible damage done to the brain by either mania or depression? What role, if any, does neuron death or birth play in mania or depression?

Note: Kindling is probably a real phenomenon that permanently predisposes the brain to future bipolar episodes.

Question 38

What is the relationship between stress and depression? What types of stress are most likely to cause depression?

Note: Stress is thought to be a cause of depression.

Question 39

Why is there diurnal fluctuation in mood during most cases of depression?

Theory: Diurnal fluctuation in mood results because the synaptic serotonin and norepinephrine levels build as the day wears on, but the postsynaptic receptor population is not saturated with the neurotransmitter. In the nondepressed individual, serotonin and norepinephrine also build as the day wears on, but the postsynaptic receptor population is already saturated.

Question 40

Does induction of mania result in reduced emotional sensitivity?

Theory: Yes.

Question 41

Is ultra-rapid cycling bipolar disorder, where mood fluctuates dramatically within one day, caused by super high norepinephrine?

Theory: Yes, since the norepinephrine system may play a role in producing emotions.

Question 42

Is there a common neurochemical basis for hallucinations that occur in some cases of depression, mania, and schizophrenia?

Theory: Yes, hallucinations only result from a very low level of serotonin.

Question 43

What aspects of our society contribute to depression?

Theory: The following aspects of American society may contribute to depression: 1) stationary and not nomadic living conditions, 2) isolated living conditions, 3) isolated working conditions, 4) unnaturally stressful working conditions, and 5) availability of too much information.

3

Other Mental Illnesses and Addictions

Question 44

What is the relationship between the Big Three neurotransmitter systems and anxiety? Is one cause of anxiety sensory overload due to low serotonin (and perhaps high norepinephrine) causing sensory-emotional hypersensitivity? Is anxiety quelled by dopamine?

Note: Cigarette smoking, which boosts the dopamine system, tends to quell anxiety. Also Zyban, which boosts dopamine and is chemically identical to Wellbutrin, is effective in helping people quit smoking.

Question 45

What is the relationship between the Big Three neurotransmitter systems and drug and alcohol abuse?

Note: Drug and alcohol abuse are common among both depressed and manic people.

Question 46

What is the relationship between the Big Three neurotransmitter systems and attention deficit hyperactivity disorder (ADHD)?

Theory: ADHD is caused by low serotonin and perhaps high norepinephrine, due to sensory-emotional hypersensitivity.

Question 47

What is the relationship between the Big Three neurotransmitter systems and the personality disorders?

Theory: Many of the personality disorders are partially caused by low serotonin.

Question 48

What is the relationship between the Big Three neurotransmitter systems and mental retardation?

Question 49

What is the relationship between the Big Three neurotransmitter systems and schizophrenia?

Note: The prevailing view is that schizophrenia is caused by excessive dopamine, since the typical antipsychotics block dopamine and terminate hallucinations.

Theory: Schizophrenia is actually caused by an abnormally low level of serotonin, since: 1) the street drug LSD, which is thought to block serotonin, produces hallucinations, 2) serotonin is distributed throughout the sensory and thinking regions of the brain, whereas dopamine is more concentrated in the thinking region of the brain, and 3) typical antipsychotics may actually raise serotonin, and thereby terminate hallucinations, through relief of negative feedback inhibition by dopamine on serotonin.

Question 50

Is mental illness a continuum or a discrete, thresholded state?

Theory: It is a continuum, with the levels of the Big Three neurotransmitters acting as continuous variables.

4

Personality

Question 51

What is the relationship between the Big Three neurotransmitter systems and personality?

Note: People are vastly different from one another, but perhaps differences in the Big Three can explain a lot of this variability, since these neurotransmitters are distributed within many different regions of the brain.

Question 52

Does the serotonin system convey the personality trait of "harm avoidance", as researcher C. Robert Cloninger has hypothesized?

Theory: Yes, but it may affect other personality traits as well.

Note: See References to find C. Robert Cloninger's personality model.

Question 53

Does the norepinephrine system convey the personality trait of "reward dependence", as researcher C. Robert Cloninger has hypothesized?

Theory: Yes, but it may affect other personality traits as well.

Note: Perhaps being high in norepinephrine causes a type of depression which is relieved in a reward dependent manner. See References to find C. Robert Cloninger's personality model.

Question 54

Does the dopamine system convey the personality trait of "novelty seeking", as researcher C. Robert Cloninger has hypothesized?

Theory: Yes, but it may affect other personality traits as well.

Note: See References to find C. Robert Cloninger's personality model.

Question 55

Does each of the Big Three neurotransmitter systems independently affect one or more personality traits, or do the Big Three interact to affect single traits?

Theory: There is no interaction of this type.

Question 56

What is the relationship between serotonin and leadership? Is the serotonin system simply designed to allow a person to achieve and maintain power, possibly by finding out what people want and delivering it? If serotonin bestows the trait of "harm avoidance", how important is it for the future welfare of this planet that our leaders be high in serotonin, since such leaders might instinctively avoid potential catastrophes?

Note: Since serotonin level correlates with social rank in animals with dominance hierarchies, serotonin may affect leadership qualities of people.

Theory: Having high serotonin leaders is critical for the future welfare of the planet.

Question 57

What is the relationship between norepinephrine and artistic temperament?

Theory: A high norepinephrine level results in sensory-emotional hypersensitivity that may be common among artists.

Question 58

Does high norepinephrine bestow a type of dominance, or at least prominence, much like high serotonin?

Theory: Many famous artists and writers have been very high in norepinephrine and low in serotonin.

Question 59

What are the characteristics of someone who is super high in serotonin and super low in norepinephrine?

Theory: Such a person is: masculine, somewhat asexual, aloof, usually skinny from lack of a strong appetite, doesn't laugh or smile much, not easily excited, harm avoidant, interested in justice, poor at tolerating the cold, adept at explosive movements, and high in energy.

Question 60

Are most of our government and big business leaders super high in serotonin?

Theory: No.

Question 61

If someone is super high in serotonin and super low in norepinephrine, and they become depressed, how should they be treated?

Theory: They should be given a norepinephrine boosting tricyclic anti-depressant, such as Desipramine or Nortriptyline. If this makes them hypomanic, a serotonin/dopamine blocking atypical antipsychotic, such as Zyprexa, should be added.

Question 62

What are the characteristics of someone who is super high in norepinephrine and super low in serotonin?

Theory: Such a person is: feminine, sexual, gregarious, strong in appetite, artistic, good at tolerating the cold, reward dependent, adept at sustained movements, and very sensitive.

Question 63

If someone is super high in norepinephrine and super low in serotonin, and they become depressed, how should they be treated?

Theory: They should be given a selective serotonin reuptake inhibitor (SSRI), such as Prozac, Zoloft, Paxil, or Celexa. If this makes them hypomanic, lithium or an anticonvulsant should be added (which I believe block norepinephrine).

Question 64

How many people have a severe excess/deficiency of one or more of the Big Three neurotransmitters? 1%, 5%, 10%, more?

Question 65

If we medicate away the extreme levels of the Big Three neurotransmitters, will we reduce high achievement, low achievement, or neither?

Question 66

What is the relationship between high achievement of any kind, mental illness, and the Big Three neurotransmitter systems?

Note: Maybe part of doing great things is to be motivated by the fact that doing medium things doesn't get a rise out of you.

Theory: Being super high in one or more of the Big Three makes high achievement more likely.

Question 67

What is the relationship between the Big Three neurotransmitter systems and nomadic behavior? Are we all naturally nomadic?

Note: Maybe in American society, the nature of our jobs keeps us in one place, but a lot of retired people drift around in RVs.

Theory: Someone who is super high in dopamine (and therefore super high in the "novelty seeking" trait, according to researcher C. Robert Cloninger) likes to move around a lot.

Question 68

Since the Big Three neurotransmitters are distributed throughout most of the brain, do they affect a variety of personality traits?

Theory: Yes.

Question 69

What is the relationship between the Big Three neurotransmitter systems and confidence?

Note: When people are manic, they tend to have grandiose thoughts about themselves, whereas depressed people tend to have highly negative thoughts about themselves.

Question 70

Does the Republican Party generally consist of high serotonin (masculine) people, and does the Democratic Party generally consist of high norepinephrine (feminine) people?

Theory: Yes, to a crude approximation.

Question 71

Does big business tend to favor high norepinephrine people, and does small business tend to favor high serotonin people?

Theory: Yes, to a crude approximation.

Question 72

Do people tend to organize themselves into social hierarchies?

Note: This is a very complex issue. Many of our social organizations, such as governments and businesses, are set up in a hierarchical fashion. However, this may have little to do with human nature, and simply is a logical way to structure large organizations.

Question 73

What does superhero worship, in books and films, indicate about human nature? Is this an instance of low serotonin people being fascinated with someone more powerful than them—i.e. someone super high in serotonin? More generally, are people skilled at identifying Big Three neurotransmitter system characteristics in others, since this may be important for social interaction?

Theory: The super high serotonin person is a natural psychologist, since understanding people is critical for achieving and maintaining power.

Question 74

Are or were the following people super high in serotonin and super low in norepinephrine (in alphabetical order): Bill Belichick, Larry Bird, Black Rob, Michael Bloomberg, Clint Eastwood, Frank Gifford, Ernest Hemingway, Ice Cube, Larry King, David Letterman, Abraham Lincoln, Kweisi Mfume, Joe Montana, Paul Newman, Mark Twain, Bill Walsh, and George Washington?

Theory: Yes.

Note: I believe this trait is much more common in men than in women, since I believe men tend to be high in serotonin and low in norepinephrine, whereas women tend to be high in norepinephrine and low in serotonin.

Question 75

Are or were the following people super high in norepinephrine and super low in serotonin (in alphabetical order): Drew Barrymore, Warren Beatty, Halle Berry, Jim Carrey, Kurt Cobain, Sheryl Crow, Tom Cruise, Robert DeNiro, Robert Downey Jr., Kay Jamison, Stephen King, John Lennon, Winona Ryder, Kevin Spacey, Steven Spielberg, Meryl Streep, and Steven Tyler?

Theory: Yes.

Note: I believe this trait is much more common among women than is super high serotonin and super low norepinephrine, since I believe women tend to be high in norepinephrine and low in serotonin, whereas men tend to be high in serotonin and low in norepinephrine.

5

Mechanisms of Existing Drugs, Treatments, and Therapy

Question 76

Do the mood stabilizers (lithium, the anticonvulsants, the atypical antipsychotics) do anything more than simply block the action of one or more of the Big Three neurotransmitters? In other words, do the mood stabilizers somehow stabilize the Big Three or just block the action of one or more of the Big Three?

Theory: Lithium and the anticonvulsants only block norepinephrine, whereas the atypical antipsychotics only block dopamine and serotonin.

Question 77

If norepinephrine plays a role in producing emotions, does blocking norepinephrine result in a type of mood stabilization, independent of and confused with stabilizing standard bipolar disorder?

Theory: Yes.

Question 78

Does Wellbutrin (a dopamine booster) exert its antidepressant effect immediately, or does it take a week or more to kick-in like the other serotonin and norepinephrine boosting antidepressants? Likewise, do the antipsychotics (dopamine blockers) exert their anti-manic effect immediately, or do they take a week or more to kick-in like lithium and the anticonvulsants?

Theory: The effect of dopamine boosting or blocking takes place immediately.

Question 79

When an antidepressant doesn't work, is it because the key doesn't fit the lock on a molecular scale (i.e. drug/receptor interaction), or is it because the key does fit the lock (neurotransmitter is boosted) but there's nothing wrong with that neurotransmitter system?

Theory: No response usually occurs because the key doesn't fit the lock on a molecular scale.

Question 80

In what instances is therapy most helpful? What types of therapy are most effective?

Theory: Cognitive therapy may be quite effective in treating mild depressions.

Question 81

Does electroconvulsive therapy (ECT) reset just one neurotransmitter system, like say norepinephrine, or does it reset each of the Big Three systems?

Theory: ECT resets each of the Big Three systems.

Question 82

Is tardive dyskinesia, a movement disorder that can result from taking antipsychotic medications, really irreversible?

Theory: Hopefully not.

Question 83

How common is medicinal adaptation? Does it just occur in certain subpopulations of patients or with certain medications? Can it be "fooled" by introducing a different drug of the same class, a drug from another class, or the same drug at a later time?

Theory: Medicinal adaptation is far less common than environmentally based retriggering of mental illness symptoms.

Question 84

Is the reason for the two-week delay in antidepressant response due to normal saturation of postsynaptic receptors (plus an extra safety factor—which means extra neurotransmitter beyond the saturation point) and the time for sprouting of new postsynaptic receptors? Is lack of saturation of the postsynaptic receptors the reason for immediate responders?

Theory: Yes, yes.

Question 85

Is there a signal present in the saliva, urine, sweat, skin, hair, feces, or blood that correlates with the level of depression or mania, or predicts response to a medication (either before or after initial administration of an antidepressant or mood stabilizer)? Is there a brain scanning technique that accomplishes these things that can be applied to the masses (i.e. for a reasonable price)?

Theory: Yes, yes.

Question 86

In the treatment of schizophrenia, do the antipsychotics (which block dopamine) work by releasing serotonin from negative feedback regulation by dopamine, thereby raising serotonin levels?

Theory: Yes.

Question 87

Does lithium affect cognition by indirectly lowering dopamine by directly lowering or blocking norepinephrine? Do the anticonvulsants also affect cognition by the same mechanism?

Theory: Yes, yes.

Note: Since dopamine is distributed heavily within the prefrontal thinking region of the brain, it's likely that it has something to do with disturbances in cognition caused by lithium.

Question 88

Does part of the confusion in the nature versus nurture debate have to do with the emotional sensitivity of a person? Is emotional sensitivity also of primary consideration in the therapy versus medications debate, with less sensitive people being less responsive to therapy?

Theory: Yes, yes.

Question 89

Is lithium just a blocker of norepinephrine, without otherwise stabilizing any neurotransmitters, and is its antidepressant effect mediated just by blocking norepinephrine?

Theory: Yes, yes.

Note: Since norepinephrine mediates the trait of "reward dependence" according to C. Robert Cloninger, perhaps blocking norepinephrine has an antidepressant effect. I would predict that the anticonvulsants, which I also postulate to be norepinephrine blockers, should also have an antidepressant effect.

Question 90

Does therapy affect brain chemistry in a way that is similar to the effect of antidepressants?

Theory: Therapy affects brain chemistry, but in a different way.

Question 91

Which effects that are direct consequences of medicinally affecting the Big Three neurotransmitter systems have been described as side effects? For example, are the sexual "side effects" of the serotonin boosting antidepressants actually direct consequences of raising serotonin?

Theory: Yes.

Question 92

Other than tardive dyskinesia, are the effects of all psychiatric medications reversible? In other words, even if there are withdrawal effects after stopping a medication, are there any permanent changes—either good or bad—that result from taking a medication?

Theory: Other than tardive dyskinesia, there are no permanent changes that the existing psychiatric medicines cause.

Question 93

Which withdrawal effects, if any, are induced by each of the psychiatric medications? How long do they typically last?

Question 94

Is polytherapy—which is use of more than one medication at a time—an intelligent strategy for treating mental illness? Can there be a synergistic effect from taking more than one medication at a time?

Note: Perhaps many different individual drugs should be tried on a given individual before more than one drug is used simultaneously.

Question 95

Are some antidepressants more effective than others? For example, can Wellbutrin (a dopamine booster) actually treat severe depression? Or at least can it make one feel better until a proper serotonin or norepinephrine booster is found?

Theory: Wellbutrin cannot treat severe depression, but can make one feel better until a proper serotonin or norepinephrine booster is found.

6

New Drugs Needed

Question 96

Should the patent duration for psychiatric medications be extended to encourage financially riskier or smaller market share drugs to be produced?

Note: Since there is a very high cost for a U.S. pharmaceutical company to bring a new drug to market (approximately 250 million dollars), companies are forced to produce drugs that they are quite confident will serve a fairly large market.

Question 97

Why is there only one dopamine booster (Wellbutrin) on the U.S. market (especially if it kicks in immediately)? The market will probably bear more than one dopamine booster due to non-responders.

Question 98

Is the latest generation of schizophrenia drugs, namely the atypical antipsychotics, very effective in treating schizophrenia?

Theory: No.

Note: Since I believe schizophrenia is caused by very low serotonin and the atypical antipsychotics block serotonin, they shouldn't be a very effective treatment. However, the atypical antipsychotics also block dopamine and may therefore be able to indirectly boost serotonin through relief of negative feedback inhibition on serotonin by dopamine.

Question 99

If one blocks serotonin with LSD and gets hallucinations, what happens when one transiently blocks norepinephrine or dopamine with some other drug?

Theory: Blocking norepinephrine will diminish the emotions, whereas blocking dopamine will diminish thinking.

Question 100

Why don't the pharmaceutical companies produce a selective serotonin blocker or a selective norepinephrine blocker?

Note: Such drugs would probably be effective in terminating mania.

References

Cloninger, C. Robert. "A Unified Biosocial Theory of Personality and Its Role in the Development of Anxiety States," *Psychiatric Developments*, vol. 3 (1986), pp. 167–226; "A Systematic Method for Clinical Description and Classification of Personality Variants: A Proposal," *Archives of General Psychiatry*, vol. 44 (1987), pp. 573–588.

Goodwin, Frederick K., Jamison Kay R. *Manic-Depressive Illness*. (Oxford: Oxford University Press, 1990).

Kramer, Peter D. *Listening to Prozac*. (New York: Viking Penguin, 1993).

Nolte, John. *The Human Brain*. (St. Louis: Mosby-Year Book, 1993).

Norden, Michael J. *Beyond Prozac*. (New York: ReganBooks, 1995).

0-595-26294-5